Asthma

All You Need To Know

Dr. Sheila Harrison

Disclaimer

This content serves to provide general information about the disease and aims to empower you to seek prompt medical assistance if necessary to prevent complications. It's essential to stress that this information is not a substitute for consulting a qualified physician. The field of medical science is continually evolving, and due to the dynamic nature of medical knowledge, we recommend seeking expert advice if you encounter any inconsistencies or intend to take action based on the information in this content. Never disregard professional medical guidance or delay treatment based on something you've read online, including this material, or from any other online source. Always remember that the internet cannot cure you; rather, healing comes through the guidance of medical professionals and the providence of God.

Table of contents

Disclaimer 2

Table of contents 3

Overview 4

Background 5

Impact OF Asthma Worldwide 8

Key facts 9

Section 1 10

    Introduction 10

Section 2 11

    Symptoms 11

Section 3 13

    Causes of Asthma 13

Section 4 15

    Asthma Triggers 15

Section 5 16

    Risk Factors 16

Section 6 17

    Types Of Asthma 17

Section 7 19

    Diagnosis 19

Section 8 21

    Medication, Treatment & Prevention 21

Overview

According to estimates from the World Health Organization (WHO), 262 million people globally experienced asthma in 2019. It has been observed that the diagnostic rates of asthma are often low, particularly in low-income countries. Asthma sufferers can have happy, fulfilling lives provided they are aware of their illness and take the necessary care of it, even though there is no known cure.

Asthma is a chronic lung illness that can strike anyone at any age. Inflammation and stiffness in the muscles surrounding the airways make breathing harder.

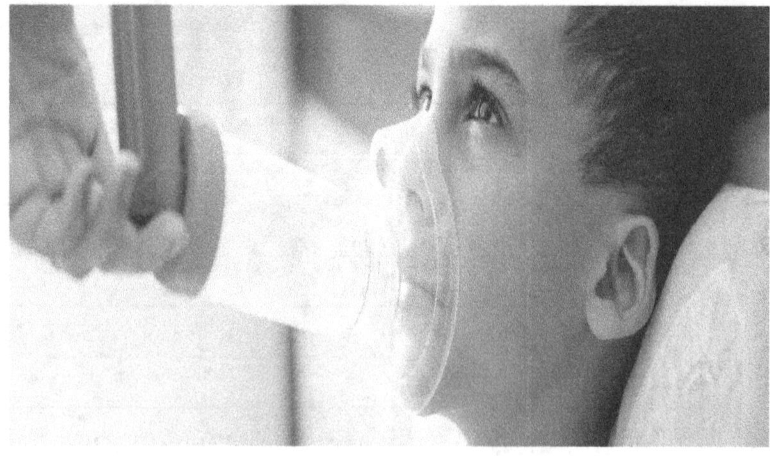

Background

A common chronic ailment worldwide, asthma affects about 26 million people in the US. It is the most common chronic illness in childhood, accounting for an estimated 6 million cases worldwide, and the primary cause of pediatric hospitalization in the United States.

The etiology of asthma is complex and involves airway inflammation, intermittent airflow limitation, and bronchial hyperresponsiveness. Apart from mucus secretion and airway edema, asthma also involves an inflammatory process that can be transient, subacute, or chronic, which worsens bronchial responsiveness and restricts airflow.

There are varying degrees of smooth muscle hyperplasia, mucus hypersecretion, desquamation of the epithelium, airway remodeling, and eosinophil and mononuclear cell infiltration. Patients with asthma who have bronchial hyperreactivity, often referred to as airway hyperresponsiveness, overreact to a range of stimuli from the environment and from within. The two processes involved are direct activation of airway smooth muscle and indirect stimulation by pharmacologically active chemicals from cells secreting mediators, like mast cells or unmyelinated sensory neurons. The degree of airway hyperresponsiveness and the intensity of asthma symptoms are usually correlated.

Spirometry using the bronchodilator response should be the main test used to confirm the diagnosis of asthma. In all individuals with acute asthma, a pulse oximetry reading is preferred in order to rule out hypoxemia. Most patients with asthma symptoms still receive a chest radiograph as their initial imaging evaluation; however, most of these individuals have normal findings on chest radiography or signals that could indicate hyperinflation. Exercise spirometry is the gold standard for diagnosing patients with bronchospasm generated by exercise.

The physical symptoms of asthma are influenced by the severity of the condition, whether an acute episode occurs, and how strong the event is. There are four categories for asthma severity: moderately persistent, severe persistent, intermittent, and mildly persistent. Depending on how bad their asthma is, people can experience mild, moderate, or severe exacerbations.

Pharmacologic management includes the use of drugs for control and alleviation. Control drugs include inhaled corticosteroids, leukotriene modifiers, leuphylline (Theo-24, Theochron, Uniphyl), long-acting bronchodilators (beta-agonists and anticholinergics), anti-IgE, anti-IL-5, and anti-IL-4/IL-13 antibodies. Painkillers include ipratropium (Atrovent), systemic corticosteroids, and short-acting bronchodilators. Depending on the severity of the exacerbation, hospitalization is recommended after a patient receives three doses of an inhaled bronchodilator. An asthma control evaluation should typically be performed on patients every one to six months.

Impact OF Asthma Worldwide

Asthma underdiagnosis and undertreatment are prevalent, particularly in low- and middle-income countries. Untreated asthma sufferers may have trouble falling asleep, feel exhausted during the day, and have trouble concentrating. Asthma sufferers may miss work or school, which can put a financial strain on the family and the community at large. If an asthmatic's symptoms are severe, they can need emergency care as well as hospital admission for treatment and monitoring. Severe asthma attacks have the potential to be deadly.

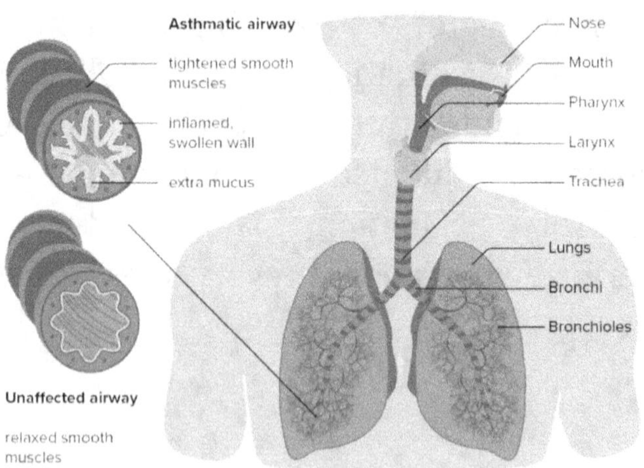

Key facts

- Asthma is a severe noncommunicable disease (NCD) that affects both adults and children, and it is the most common chronic illness in children.
- The inflammation and constriction of the lungs' narrow airways cause asthma symptoms, which can include any combination of cough, wheeze, shortness of breath, and tightness in the chest.
- With inhaled medication, people with asthma can maintain normal, active lifestyles while controlling their symptoms.
- Asthma symptoms can be lessened by reducing asthma triggers.
- Most deaths from asthma occur in low- and lower-middle-income countries, where individuals can be challenging to detect and treat.
- As part of its mission to reduce the global burden of NCDs and advance universal health coverage, WHO is committed to improving asthma diagnosis, treatment, and surveillance.

Section 1

Introduction

Asthma is an inflammatory disease that causes the airways to become extremely sensitive to a trigger. Constriction of the airways and inflammation make breathing difficult. Inhaling air purifies blood as it passes through the trachea and airways into the lungs of a healthy individual. These airways have cilia that secrete mucus and smooth muscles along their walls. Cilia stop dust from getting into the airways.

The severity of the condition might range from mild to very severe. In the early stages, the patient has infrequent asthma attacks; nevertheless, by the latter stages, their quality of life has considerably declined.

During an asthma attack, these smooth muscles swell and become inflamed, causing the cilia to oversecrete mucus and block the airways.

The following are the causes of an asthma attack:

1. Tightening of the muscles that line the airways

2. Increased mucus secretion

3. Inflammation of airways

Section 2

Symptoms

Asthma can be a dangerous illness, but it can also be treated with the right care. People who are having symptoms of asthma should see a physician. Among the symptoms include chest tightness, wheezing, coughing, and shortness of breath. These symptoms could get worse or better with time.

The symptoms of asthma might vary from person to person. Occasionally, the symptoms suddenly get worse. This is known as an asthma attack. Symptoms frequently get worse at night or during exercising.

Common symptoms of asthma include:
- A chronic cough, particularly at night.
- Wheezing occasionally during inhalation and exhalation.
- Breathing difficulties or shortness of breath, occasionally even at rest.

- Chest constriction, which makes deep breathing challenging.
- Cough
- Trouble falling asleep.
- Recurring respiratory illnesses.
- Agitation.
- Difficulty conversing and working out.
- Attacks that happen at specific times (nocturnal), while working, or during an activity (exercise induced)

Some persons experience worsening symptoms when they have a cold or when the temperature drops. Other triggers include animal fur and feathers, harsh soaps, smoking, dust, fumes, pollen from grasses and trees, and scent.

The symptoms may also be brought on by certain illnesses. Individuals who exhibit symptoms should see a doctor.

Section 3

Causes of Asthma

There is currently no proven cause for asthma, despite the fact that a number of factors have been linked to an increased chance of developing the condition and that it is usually difficult to pinpoint a single, direct cause. The literature now in publication shows that the disease's development is impacted by both environmental and genetic factors.

1. **Genetic factors:** Numerous genes have been connected to heightened vulnerability to asthma risk factors. Other family members who also have asthma, especially close relatives like parents or siblings, increase the likelihood of developing asthma.

2. **Environmental factors:** The environment contains a variety of compounds known as allergens that irritate the airways. Inflammation results from the mucosa secreting different molecules, such as interleukins, in response to contact with the allergen.

Eczema and rhinitis (hay fever) are among the other allergic disorders that might arise. Asthma risk is also believed to be increased by exposure to a variety of environmental allergens and irritants, such as mold, indoor and outdoor air pollution, dust mites in the home, and dust, fumes, and chemicals in the workplace.

3. **Urbanization:** The prevalence of asthma is known to rise with urbanization, most likely as a result of various lifestyle variables.

4. **Life Style:** Early life experiences have an impact on the developing lungs and can raise the likelihood of acquiring asthma. Prematurity, low birth weight, exposure to tobacco smoke and other air pollution sources, and viral respiratory infections are a few of these.

5. **Obesity:** Obese or overweight individuals and children are more likely to develop asthma.

Section 4

Asthma Triggers

The most common triggers/environmental allergens have been listed below:

1. Pollen
2. Dust
3. Fungal spores
4. Pet fur
5. Cold air
6. Smoke
7. Exercise
8. Medicines like aspirin, ibuprofen, beta blockers
9. Air pollutants
10. Emotional stress
11. Gastroesophageal reflux disease
12. Preservatives added in the food
13. Food allergens like prawns, peanuts

Section 5

Risk Factors

1. **Obesity:** It raises the likelihood of contracting the illness.

2. **Hygiene hypothesis:** According to the theory, overprotecting kids from dust and other allergens outside of their bodies causes the mucosal wall of their respiratory system to become hypersensitive when they are eventually exposed to them.

3. **History of other allergic diseases**: A person's immune system may be triggered by previous allergy disorders such as rhinitis and eczema, which increases the likelihood of developing asthma.

4. **Viral infections:** It has been demonstrated that a positive history of Respiratory Syncytial Virus (RSV) infection causes asthma in later life.

Section 6

Types Of Asthma

1. **Childhood Asthma:** These are extremely early-life asthma attacks, usually linked to genetics or a family history of allergies.

2. **Adolescent Asthma:** Usually caused by a history of viral illness, the child's symptoms initially appear throughout puberty.

3. **Occupational Asthma:** The symptoms are linked to a particular industry where the worker is exposed to inflammatory allergens, such as the rubber, dye, or petrochemical sectors.

4. **Seasonal Asthma:** The symptoms only worsen at certain seasons of the year, such as the spring when pollen is in the air. Pollen may act as an asthma attack trigger in several conditions.

5. **Physical activity-induced Asthma:** Normally, dust is removed from air before it reaches the lungs as it enters the respiratory system. However, during

exercise, people tend to breathe more rapidly and often via their mouths. Consequently, there is no filtering of the air that reaches the lungs.

6. **Aspirin-induced asthma:** In this type, consuming drugs like ibuprofen or aspirin could result in an asthma attack..

7. **Asthma that flares up at night:** At night, this type of asthma flares up or gets worse.

8. **Variant of cough Asthma:** Mucus is not secreted by this species. There is a long-lasting, persistent dry cough that, if addressed, can turn into severe asthma.

Section 7

Diagnosis

The following tests are done in order to make the diagnosis:

1. **Family history:** It's taken in order to know the prevalence of asthma in the family.

2. **Allergic history:** History for any other hypersensitivity present in the individual.

3. **Physical examination:** It is done to diagnose asthma by listening to lungs for wheezing, examining the nose and throat for swelling and checking for barrel-shaped chest, which is common among kids suffering from childhood asthma.

4. **Patch test:** In this, triggering allergens are identified by putting various allergens in contact with the skin and checking the sensitivity against each.

5. **Chest X-ray:** In the cases of severe asthmatic attacks, a doctor may suggest

a chest X-ray. Chest X-rays also help in diagnosing lung or heart diseases among asthma patients who exhibit their symptoms.

6. **Pulmonary function test:** Various lung capacities like inhalation and exhalation are checked, which gets affected in the cases of asthma.

7. **Blood tests:** To check the levels of immunoglobulin E, which increases in the cases of hypersensitivity diseases like asthma.

Section 8

Medication, Treatment & Prevention

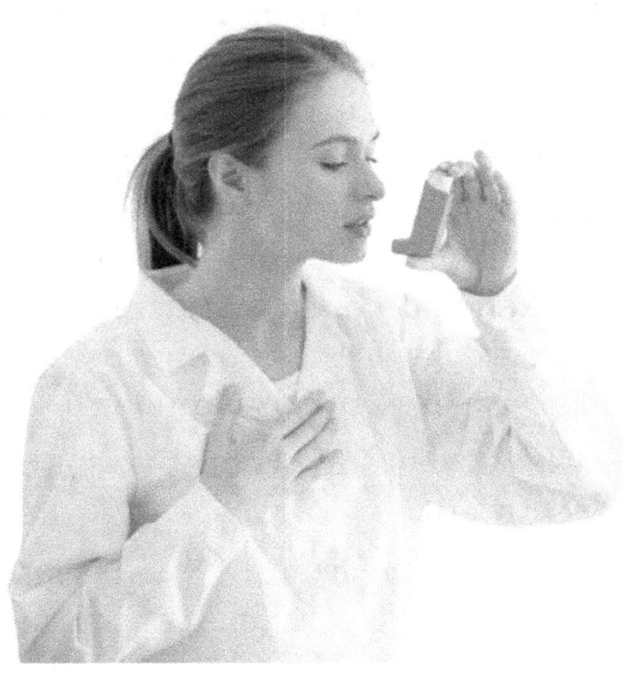

Pharmaceutical supervision/Control

Generally speaking, there are two kinds of asthma medications based on whether we are addressing a long-term strategy or acute asthma attack:

1. **Treatment for acute attack / Quick relief (also called reliever medications):**

Quick relief medications are used to ease acute asthma exacerbations and to prevent exercise-induced bronchoconstriction (EIB) symptoms. These medications speed up the healing process after acute exacerbations and include salbutamol, a short-acting beta agonist (SABA), and systemic corticosteroids. can be given under the doctors' observation. Acute inflammation decrease is achieved with the use of steroids like beclomethasone. Inhalers are used to give these two medications.

2. **Long term preventative / Control treatment:**

Leukotriene antagonists and mast cell stabilizers are two examples of drugs that can be used to prevent the release of inflammatory substances. Medications used for long-term management include inhalation corticosteroids (ICSs), long-acting beta agonists (LABAs) [102, 103], long-acting anticholinergics, combination inhaled corticosteroids and long-acting beta agonists, methylxanthines, and leukotriene receptor antagonists. While inhaled corticosteroids are generally considered the first-choice drug for treating chronic asthma, the response to this treatment varies sadly throughout patients.

There are several treatments for asthma, however there is yet no cure for the condition. Direct inhalation of medication into the lungs is the most common treatment method.

Asthmatics can live regular, active lives and better manage their condition by using inhalers. There are primarily two kinds of inhalers:

- Bronchodilators (such as salbutamol), that open the air passages and relieve symptoms; and

- Steroids (such as beclometasone) that reduce inflammation in the air passages, which improves asthma symptoms and reduces the risk of severe asthma attacks and death.

People who have asthma may need to take their inhaler on a daily basis. Treatment for them will depend on how often they experience symptoms and what kind of inhalers are available.

Using an inhaler can be difficult, especially for little children or in an emergency. Using a spacer device makes using an aerosol inhaler easier. This makes it easier for the drug to enter the lungs and absorb. A spacer is a plastic device with a mouthpiece or mask on one end and an inhaler hole on the other. You can create an affordable, handcrafted spacer that works just as well as ones you can buy in stores using a 500 ml plastic bottle.

In many countries, it is difficult to obtain inhalers. In 2021, bronchodilators were available in half of low- and low-middle-income countries, while steroid inhalers were available in a third of public primary health care institutions. Increasing community knowledge is also essential to eradicating the stigma and myths surrounding asthma in specific circumstances.

Salbutamol

Beclometasone

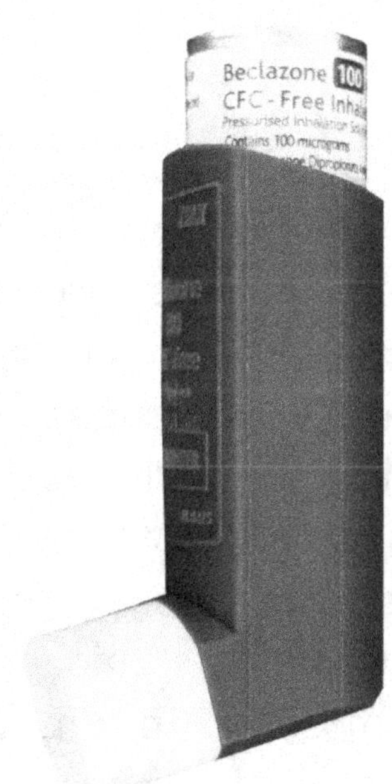

Self-care

Those who have asthma and their family need to be educated so they may understand more about their condition. This includes what triggers to stay away from, therapies that are currently accessible, and at-home symptom management.

It is critical for people to understand when to boost their therapy when their symptoms worsen in order to avoid a disastrous asthma attack. Medical practitioners may provide patients an asthma action plan so they can better control their asthma.

Environmental Control

Exposure to environmental irritants can have a substantial impact on the worsening of symptoms. Therefore, in individuals with persistent asthma, it is crucial to assess susceptibility to long-term indoor allergens using in vitro testing or skin testing. Once the allergens causing the issue have been determined, provide patients guidance on how to prevent these exposures. Information about preventing exposure to secondhand and firsthand tobacco smoke is also beneficial for asthma patients.

There are a number of strategies to stay away from any particular allergen, depending on its size and properties. As soon as an allergy is avoided, symptoms should usually go away fairly fast; nevertheless, the allergen itself (cat dander, for example) may stay in the air for months after the source is initially eliminated. Single efforts rarely succeed on their own, necessitating a holistic plan.

Comprehensive allergen avoidance during the first year of life considerably delays the onset of asthma in persons with a high hereditary risk; the impact appears early in childhood and persists into adulthood.

The house is where you should spend the most of your time—between thirty and sixty percent. Regular cleaning and dusting should be done in the homes of patients. If patients are unable to avoid vacuuming, they should wear a face mask or a double-bagged vacuum with a high-efficiency particle air filter. If at all possible, moving to a higher floor of the house (less dust and mold) or to a new neighborhood (fewer cockroaches) may be considered. It is essential that you refrain from smoking, both actively and passively.

Room air ionizers have not been demonstrated to help persons with persistent asthma, and the ozone these devices produce may be harmful to some people. Certain factors associated to the home include dust mites, animals, cockroaches, mold, and pollen (for further details, see Indoor Aeroallergens).

Air pollution from traffic can increase the risk of wheezing and asthma, especially in those with high EPHX1 gene and enzyme activity. By causing oxidative stress in the airways, this might be mediated.

Dust mites

The primary allergen for dust mites (Dermatophagoides pteronyssinus and farina, size 30 μm) is an intestinal enzyme on fecal particles. The allergen sits on fabric, making air filtering ineffective because of its relatively large size. One method of preventing dust mites is to use impermeable covers (the most significant intervention, for mattresses, pillows, and comforters). Another is to remove rugs from beds, limit upholstered furniture, reduce the amount of window blinds, wash other bedding in hot water (130°F [54.4°C] is the most effective temperature), and store clothes in drawers and closets. Cut down on the number of stuffed animals you own, and either give them a weekly wash or occasionally put them in the freezer. Cut the humidity in the room to under 50%.

Because cat and other animal dander, saliva, urine, and serum proteins are so small (1–20 μm), most of these allergens are airborne indoor allergens. Avoidance tactics include removing animals from the house—or at least the bedroom—and cleaning cats and dogs up to twice a week, as well as blocking heating and cooling duct vents with dense filtering material. Cat antigen has been found in homes and workplaces where cats have never lived, highlighting the importance of regular cleaning. Even after cats are gone from a home, the antigens can persist there for up to six months.

Allergen Immunotherapy

Whether immunotherapy is appropriate for treating asthma is up for debate. The effectiveness of the treatment for asthma was confirmed by a meta-analysis of 75 randomized controlled trials, even though some large, meticulously conducted research yielded negative findings.

The National Asthma Education and Prevention Program's Expert Panel Report states that immunotherapy should be considered when the following circumstances are met:

- There is little question that the patient's sensitivity to an inevitable allergen and the symptoms are related.
- The symptoms are present for a considerable portion of the year or the entire year.
- When a patient is not adhering to their pharmaceutical regimen, requires many medications, or is taking inefficient medication, pharmacologic management of symptoms can be difficult.

Recurrent injections of tiny quantities of allergen have been used to treat allergic rhinitis for more than a century. Benefits may remain for years after treatment is stopped, indicating how clearly successful the treatment is. This drug is also considered required for reactions to wasp and bee venom (hymenoptera) that could be lethal. The importance of repeated allergen injections in asthma patients has been more contentious, with views ranging from a relative indication to none at all. Benefits have been demonstrated in individuals with allergy-induced asthma.

Monoclonal Antibody Therapy

Omalizumab is advised for adults and children aged six or older with moderate-to-severe persistent asthma whose symptoms are not well controlled with inhaled corticosteroids when a skin test yields a positive result or an in vitro reactivity to a perennial aeroallergen is obtained. IgE levels should range from 30 to 700 IU, and weights should not exceed 150 kg.

This is a humanized murine IgG antibody that targets the Fc portion of the IgE antibody, which clings to mast cell surfaces. This antibody inhibits mast cell receptor-mediated IgE attachment, hence preventing mast cell degranulation without inducing degranulation itself.

Bronchial Thermoplasty

A series of bronchoscopy techniques are used to provide regulated thermal energy to the airway wall during bronchial thermoplasty (BT), a new asthma intervention.

Asthma in Pregnancy

Asthma causes pregnancy complications in 4-8% of cases. When mild asthma is appropriately managed, results for mothers and perinatals during pregnancy can be great. Severe and poorly controlled asthma may increase the risk of preterm birth and other perinatal issues, such as mother morbidity and mortality. Pregnancy-related asthma is best treated with patient education, individualized pharmaceutical medication, objective lung function monitoring, and minimizing or eliminating asthma triggers. Inhaled corticosteroids are the recommended treatment for all severity levels of chronic asthma during pregnancy. Medicating pregnant women with asthma is a safer option than letting the condition worsen and causing symptoms to worsen. The ultimate goal of asthma therapy is to prevent hypoxic episodes in the mother in order to maintain the fetus's normal oxygenation.

Approach to Level of Activity

Patients' level of activity is typically restricted by their ability to exercise and how they respond to medicine. While there are no specific guidelines for patients with asthma, it is advisable for them to avoid anything that can aggravate their disease.

Maintaining baseline asthma therapy should be able to prevent exertional symptoms, as many asthma patients also experience exercise-induced bronchoconstriction. Individuals with exercise-induced bronchoconstriction may or may not be able to exercise, depending on their fitness level, the kind of exercise they perform, and the environment in which they exercise. Many patients report fewer problems when exercising indoors or in a warm, humid environment than when they exercise outside or in a cold, dry one.

Dietary Considerations

Evidence from prospective cohort studies and population-based research undertaken in the past few years suggests a link between obesity and asthma. People with greater body mass indices are more prone to asthma. In the Nurses' Health trial II, a prospective cohort trial involving around 86,000 adult women, a five-year observation period showed a linear relationship between body mass index and the risk of developing asthma. Obese asthma patients had more comorbidities and a worse lung function than normal-weight asthma patients, according to the 2019 GINA recommendation. Patients who are obese may find it more difficult to manage their asthma; nevertheless, a 5–10% weight loss can improve asthma control and quality of life.

Generally speaking, no particular diet is suggested. Asthma episodes are not usually brought on by food sensitivities. Milk-containing products don't always need to be avoided unless a specific sensitivity is clearly present. After a double-blind food challenge with positive results, food avoidance is recommended. Those who are sensitive to sulfites should stay away from them because they have been connected to severe exacerbations of asthma.

Gastroesophageal Reflux Disease

Acid in the distal esophagus can dramatically increase airway resistance and sensitivity through vagal or other neural responses. Asthma is three times as common in those with GERD. At [16] Aggressive antireflux therapy may improve lung function and lessen asthma symptoms in certain patients. An inexplicable chronic cough or symptoms of asthma can be treated with proton pump inhibitors, antacids, or H2 blockers.

The esophageal sphincter's tone is decreased when theophylline or other asthma drugs are used, which may result in GERD symptoms. Some asthmatics experience significant reflux of the stomach even when they don't have any symptoms of the esophagus.

Sinusitis

50% of people who have asthma also have nasal issues. Sinusitis is the primary factor contributing to worsening asthma symptoms. Worsening symptoms of the airways could be brought on by an acute infectious sinus infection or persistent inflammation. Treatment for nasal and sinus inflammation reduces airway responsiveness. For acute sinusitis to be treated and asthma symptoms to be reduced, antibiotics must be taken for a minimum of 10 days.

Long-Term Monitoring

The following criteria should be used for ongoing monitoring of all asthma patients in order to aid in the overall management of the condition:

- Patients should be trained to identify insufficient asthma control, and healthcare professionals should evaluate control at every visit in order to monitor asthma signs and symptoms.

- Spirometry and peak-flow monitoring should be done on a frequent basis to keep an eye on lung function.

- Ask about reduced activities, sleep disruptions, missing work or school days, and changes in caregiver responsibilities in order to assess quality of life and functional status.

- In order to keep track of the history of asthma exacerbations, find out if patients are keeping an eye on themselves to identify asthma exacerbations and if they are being treated by medical professionals or on their own

- Ensure that short-acting beta agonists are used as prescribed and that medication compliance is monitored when it comes to pharmacotherapy.

- Keep an eye on patient satisfaction and provider-patient communication.

Functional Assessment of Airway Obstruction

As part of a functional assessment of airway blockage, measure the FEV1 or peak expiratory flow (PEF) to see how well the patient is responding to treatment. PEF measurement is inexpensive and portable. Serial measurements can be used to monitor a patient's response to therapy and other pertinent factors when deciding whether to admit them to the hospital or discharge them from the emergency room. One of the disadvantages of PEF is its dependence on patient work. FEV1 is more exertion-dependent than PEF.

Consultations

- Refer any patient with moderate-to-severe persistent asthma that is difficult to control to a pulmonologist or allergist to ensure appropriate stepwise asthma management. Additionally, you can refer them for further evaluation in order to assist rule out other illnesses such as VCD/ILO. A professional referral for further evaluation ought to follow any anomalies found during a chest radiography screening.

- Refer patients to an allergist or immunologist for skin testing to aid in indoor allergen avoidance and immunotherapy consideration for managing seasonal allergic rhinitis.
- Individuals who exhibit signs of exercise-induced bronchoconstriction (EIB) ought to be sent to a pulmonologist for evaluation. These patients should be given exercise or bronchoprovocation tests so that any evidence of airway hyperreactivity can be noted, as well as how the patients respond to the exercise.
- Refer patients to an otolaryngologist for the diagnosis of upper airway illnesses or for the management of nasal obstruction brought on by polyps, sinusitis, or allergic rhinitis.

Prevention Summary

The following ways can help to minimize attacks and to identify them early on:

1. Avoid triggering allergens.

2. Follow the asthma medications regimen seriously.

3. Get vaccinated with the latest flu shots.

4. Avoid smoking

5. Maintain a healthy weight

6. Have a good diet

7. In case of exercise induced asthma, avoid rigorous working out.

8. In case of occupational asthma, try to change the profession.

9. Monitor your breathing rate and sound.